Pain-Free Periods:

Yes, It Is Possible!

Mary Louise

© Copyright 2021 – Mary Louise; All rights reserved.

Scripture quotations marked (NKJV) are taken from the New King James Version®. Copyright © 1982 by Thomas Nelson. Used by permission. All rights reserved.

Scripture quotations marked (NLT) are taken from the Holy Bible, New Living Translation, copyright ©1996, 2004, 2015 by Tyndale House Foundation. Used by permission of Tyndale House Publishers, Inc., Carol Stream, Illinois 60188. All rights reserved.

Printed in the United States of America

ISBN 978-1-7375710-4-9

Contents

Getting Pain-Free   5

Helpful Scripture References   29

Other Titles by this Author   31

Getting Pain-Free

How many women would like to get rid of period pain? How many men would like the women in their lives to not suffer each month?

I suffered from horrible period pain for over twenty years; then, God showed me that I didn't have to anymore. For more than three years, I've been free from period pain. God showed me that I have authority over pain.

Eight steps enabled me to get rid of period pain. The first 7 apply to getting rid of any type of pain.

Do you have any pain in your body that you would like to get rid of?

Steps to getting rid of period pain:
1. Have a personal relationship with Jesus.
2. Change your mindset.
3. Stop accepting the pain.
4. Face the pain.
5. Fast at the onset of the pain.
6. Use your authority and tell the pain and Satan to leave in Jesus' name.
7. Refuse to believe or accept symptoms over God's Words.
8. Change the products you are using.

Pain-Free Periods: Yes, It Is Possible!

The first step is to have a personal relationship with Jesus. If I didn't have this, I wouldn't have learned that I have authority over pain.

God, the Creator of the universe, loves us very much. He sent His only Son Jesus to pay the price and penalty for our sins.

Jesus, the sinless Son of God, left heaven, came to earth, and paid the price for our sins. He allowed all the sins of the world to be put upon Him on a cross. He died a cruel death for you and for me.

Jesus didn't just die on a cross though. He rose again on the third day. When He overcame death, He enabled us to overcome anything in this life through Him.

When I asked Jesus to forgive my sins and to come into my heart, He did. And when He did, His Spirit came to live inside me. This is often referred to as salvation. We are saved from the penalty of our sins.

This is how my personal relationship with Jesus began. Jesus loved me when I was at my worst. He is so full of grace and mercy. He is loving and kind. He is the best friend that I have ever had.

Those who have a personal relationship with Jesus have no barrier of the penalty of their sins preventing them from accessing a holy and sinless God. We also now have eternal life with God and Jesus in heaven after we leave this earth.

If you haven't yet asked Jesus into your heart, now is the perfect time. If you believe that He died and rose again for you and for me, take a moment to let Him know that.

"Jesus, I believe that You died on a cross for my sins. Please forgive me for my sins of _____." Take some time to list those sins to Him. "Cleanse me, and come into my heart." It's as simple as that.

The second step to getting rid of period pain is to change your mindset. The problem with the mindset regarding period pain is that many women expect their periods to be horrible. They believe that painful periods are their lot in life that they must suffer through indefinitely. They know that other women have suffered from this, so they believe that they also must suffer. I used to have this mindset.

This mindset that women have some kind of a curse that they must suffer through each month during their period is a lie from the pit of hell. Jesus took all sickness and pain onto His body on the cross so that we don't have to. According to Isaiah 53:5, NKJV, complete healing is our inheritance as children of God. "But He was wounded for our transgressions, He was bruised for our iniquities; The chastisement for our peace was upon Him, And by His stripes we are healed."

This means that total healing and freedom from all pain, including period pain, is available to us. Jesus not only had all of the pain of the world put upon Him, but He also overcame it all when He rose from the dead. That same power to overcome all pain and death is now available to us through His Spirit. Jesus' Spirit lives inside all who have a personal relationship with Him.

Some specific things happened that showed me that I have authority over pain.

I was driving home one night when suddenly, I had this piercing pain in my abdomen. It was a pain unlike any I had ever felt. It wasn't a nauseous feeling, and it wasn't menstrual pain. It felt overwhelming and debilitating. It seemed to come out of nowhere. I immediately sensed that this was not just a physical thing that was happening; it was also spiritual.

God had been showing me to take authority over things that try to come to me that aren't from Him. Jesus tells us in John 10:10, NLT, how to test whether something is from God or Satan. "The thief's purpose is to steal and kill and destroy. My purpose is to give them a rich and satisfying life."

This pain was not helping me have a rich and satisfying life, so I knew that it wasn't from Jesus. That left one other option: Satan, the thief.

In Matthew 4:10, NLT, Jesus gives us an example of what to do when dealing with Satan. Jesus told him, "Get out of here, Satan." So, being silent with this pain from Satan wasn't an option. I started commanding the pain and Satan to leave in Jesus' name.

If you've never talked out loud to something that you can't see, it might feel strange at first. But, the more you do it, the more comfortable you will get with it. The first time you do something is usually the hardest.

Although I had told the pain and Satan to leave, the pain in my abdomen persisted. It was so bad that I almost pulled my car over to the side of the road. I could barely sit up enough to continue driving.

Fearful thoughts came at me. "What if it's a stroke?" "What if your gall bladder is about to burst?" "Maybe you should rush yourself to the emergency room."

Thoughts can come from 3 sources: God, Satan, or ourselves. The thoughts that came to me that caused me to contemplate rushing to the emergency room were rooted in fear. II Timothy 1:7, NKJV, says that God does not give us a spirit of fear. Since the fear is not coming from myself, this leaves one culprit: Satan.

So, I've determined that the pain and the thoughts that want me to rush to the emergency room are both from Satan. But, the pain and the symptoms that I feel are real, so, what do I do?

I felt that I needed to stand my ground, so I drove home instead of going to the emergency room. I chose faith instead of fear.

When I got home, it was difficult to get out of the car because of the pain. With great effort, I made it inside. All I wanted to do was lie down, but I heard God say, "When you're in a battle, the last thing that you do is lie down."

So, I stood up in my kitchen and battled this thing that was attacking my body and my mind. Although this was happening in the natural, there was something spiritual and unseen behind it, so I started using spiritual weapons.

I quoted every applicable Scripture that I could think of. "I am healed by the wounds of Jesus" (Isaiah 53:5). "Greater is He that is in me than he that is in the world" (I John 4:4). "No weapon that forms against me will prosper" (Isaiah 54:17). I also quoted parts of the spiritual armor mentioned in Ephesians 6 that I could remember. "I hold up the shield of faith. I put on the breastplate of righteousness. I wear the belt of truth."

The pain continued; it wasn't lessening. But I knew that I must fight, so that's what I did.

I continued to talk to God as I fought this battle. I was in great pain. God put on my heart to put some praise and worship music on, so I did.

When I least felt like praising, I praised and worshipped God. I also continued to tell Satan and the pain to go. I continued to quote Scripture too.

I sensed from God that I should war against this until after midnight. After over an hour, midnight came. Although the pain had lessened some, it was still pretty intense.

I sensed from God that it was now ok to go to bed. This required a lot of trust.

Pain-Free Periods: Yes, It Is Possible!

Something is definitely still going on inside my body, yet, I'm going to go to bed?

I did go to bed. Guess what happened. I slept fine that night, and the next morning when I woke up, the pain was completely gone! Hallelujah!

What might have happened if I had accepted this pain? What would have happened if I had rushed to the emergency room? My guess is that they would have seen whatever this was that the devil was slinging my way and then would've wanted to take some serious action.

Satan is real, and he is out to steal, kill, and destroy (John 10:10). He's currently loose in the world and is influencing many things. Although he is unseen, the effects of what he is up to often can be seen and felt.

Satan had come to me with symptoms that he hoped I would act on. He hoped that I would accept the symptoms. He also hoped that I would yield to fear and run to the emergency room. He hoped that I would allow them to x-ray me, find whatever it was he was inflicting upon me, and then give me a bad diagnosis. He hoped that I would accept the bad diagnosis and any proposed treatment. Maybe he hoped to take one of my organs in the process. Maybe he wanted to have access to my body to infect me with something if I allowed them to cut me open and supposedly "help" me.

The devil hopes that we will yield to fear instead of faith. He also hopes that we will not fight back and will accept whatever he sends to us as if we have no say-so or authority in the matter.

I have learned that sometimes, we have something because we say that we have it. Our words have power and bring about things. Our words bring "fruit." According to Proverbs 18:21, NKJV, the tongue has the power of life and death.

For instance, I used to believe and say that I was allergic to pollen. I believed this since I seemed to sneeze around it. God showed me that I needed to stop believing and stop speaking that I was allergic to pollen. I also needed to stop writing that I was allergic to it on forms at doctors' offices.

Once I stopped claiming that I had a pollen allergy and stopped taking medication for it, the symptoms of being allergic began to dissipate. And in a short time, the symptoms stopped completely. I no longer had any more reactions to pollen. I was no longer allergic.

Pain-Free Periods: Yes, It Is Possible!

Our mindsets and our words are important.

It's important to not listen to symptoms over God's Words. Again, we are healed by Jesus' wounds. He paid the price so that we don't have to.

It's also important to not speak that you have something, unless it is something that you actually want to have. What have you been claiming that you have?

What symptoms did you come into agreement with? It's not too late to stop claiming and stop believing those symptoms or that diagnosis. It's not too late to stand up to that thing and command it to leave you in Jesus' name.

You must be careful to not accept a diagnosis that says that you have anything other than perfect health. Although you had symptoms from the devil, if you accept a diagnosis and say that you have something, you really will have it. Your words will bring fruit.

Our agreement and our words have power and authority. The devil wants our agreement and our words. Be careful what you say.

Sometimes, we have accepted things because almost everyone else seems to. That is not a good reason.

Getting Pain-Free

And just because the medical community has an explanation or a name for something, that does not mean that we have to accept it or come into agreement with it. Our bodies are temples of the Holy Spirit.

Everything must bow at the name of Jesus (Philippians 2:9-11). This includes cancer, period pain, aids, diabetes, high blood pressure, etc. Jesus is the name above every name. Just because the devil gave the medical community a name for certain symptoms, that does not mean that that name is over the name of Jesus.

Since I have authority over other types of pain and am telling them to go, why was I accepting period pain? God showed me that I needed to **stop accepting it**.

I also needed to stop expecting that my period was going to be bad or painful. Up to this point, the first 1½ days of my period were usually horrible. I could barely function during that time. Sometimes, I would double over in misery.

I found that putting food in my system seemed to make the pain worse, but even if I ate less or didn't eat, the pain didn't go away by any means.

Basically, it was a matter of getting

through those first two days of my period. Two days can be a long time when one is in misery and excruciating pain.

At some point, I had discovered that I could cover up the horrible pain if I took a certain pain reliever medication every three to four hours. I had to take more than the recommended dosage in order to stay ahead of the pain.

Now, I needed to make a choice to face the pain and not rely on the pills. So, by faith, I threw all of the pain reliever pills in the garbage.

The next month, my period came, and the pain came along with it. God led me to not eat anything that day while I was standing up to the pain, so I fasted, along with the next steps.

I told the pain that it was not welcome here, and I commanded it go in Jesus' name. I also commanded Satan to leave. Then, I had to mean what I said. I needed to continue to stand my ground and not give in or give up even if the pain didn't leave immediately. I needed to stand my ground for however long it took.

The pain did not go away immediately. In fact, there was about an hour or more of

Getting Pain-Free

horrendous pain. It was as if Satan was trying to make it worse because I was choosing to stand up to him and not back down.

I stood up at my desk and moved around a bit because the pain was worse when I sat still. I also felt like God wanted me to literally stand up to the pain, so I did. The first hour was horrible. Every minute felt like an eternity.

Satan is persistent. He hopes that he will outlast us and that we will give up easily. That's how he has gotten away with a lot. People haven't stood up to him and stood their ground for however long it takes.

I refuse to accept anything less than what God's Word says about me as a believer. By Jesus' wounds, I am healed, period. I don't accept anything else.

With God's help, I persevered and pressed in. Within two hours, most of the pain was gone! This was huge! Although there was some discomfort after that, there was very little pain. And the rest of that week was a total breeze. Wow!

I have now covered steps two through seven of how to get rid of pain. There was one more important step though to fully get rid of period pain.

Pain-Free Periods: Yes, It Is Possible!

Before the next month came, God led me to some other pertinent information. One revelation, if we walk in it, tends to lead to the next revelation. God had me thinking about the products that I was using during my period.

First, God changed my thinking about tampons. I've heard that some women have more pain during their periods when they use tampons. I hadn't considered that tampons could be part of the problem. I had used them for so long, as I had thought that they were cleaner and more discreet.

I don't remember if I had as much pain when my cycles first started and I wasn't using tampons. Using something to stop up what our bodies are trying to naturally release is something to think about.

God then led me to research cloth pads online. Most of the cloth pads that I found advertised that they were made from natural materials.

I looked at the packages of disposable pads in stores, and most of them don't even tell you what all is in them. Hmm.

The more I learned about cloth pads and about those who had switched from disposable pads and tampons to natural, cloth pads, the more I knew that I had to try cloth pads. God then prompted me to get rid of all of my disposable tampons and pads, so I did.

I went online and ordered some cloth pads made only from the natural materials of hemp and cotton. I was even able to pick out my favorite fabric and color choice to have on the outside of the cloth pads.

The cloth pads arrived before my next period came. Strangely, I found that I was excited about using these new pads. I had never been excited in any way about anything connected to my period, yet, simply changing the products that I was using seemed to shift my mindset and my feelings about my period without any conscious effort.

My period in month two of standing up to period pain started this morning. I could feel in my body that my cycle was underway. I put on one of my new, cloth pads and packed some to bring to work. I felt led to avoid breads and foods rich in carbohydrates, so I mostly ate protein. I also made a point to not eat too much.

As the morning progressed, I felt some discomfort and pain. I told it to leave in Jesus' name. Then, I found myself welcoming my cycle. In my own way and in my own words, I actually told my body that I was not going to fight what it needed to do and was created to do.

I think that this is part of the problem with tampons. They work against what a woman's body is naturally meant to do. A woman's body is supposed to release the blood, not keep it stopped up inside for many hours.

There was discomfort part of the morning. I told all discomfort that it was not welcome and that it had to go in Jesus' name. I only experienced pain maybe two times. I resisted the pain and told it to leave when it tried to come, and it left! There was definitely no excruciating pain, and I did not need to stand up at my desk. I didn't even think about pain medication.

I realized how at peace I was and how I was having no pain during the time that was always the worst part. It's hard to explain how much joy this brings me.

Putting a material up against my body that is natural, comfortable, and chemical-free makes such a huge difference. I hadn't realized that the other materials weren't comfortable or that they were negatively affecting me because they were all I had ever known.

Getting Pain-Free

I'm not even 24 hours into my period, and I can't help but be excited. Those are words that I never thought I would say about my period.

I realized that I had been despising my own body and the process that God made. I also had been disconnected from my period through tampons and pain medication. I didn't really have to see what my body was going through with tampons or fully feel it because of the pain medication.

If a woman is not used to seeing what naturally comes out of her body during this time, there is a point of even choosing to accept the visual aspect of this God-made process that enables reproduction.

I'm in day one, when my body typically releases the most fluid. I just went to the restroom and did something that I don't usually do. I smelled my bodily fluid. There was literally zero odor or unpleasant smell from this cloth pad and my bodily fluid. I've been using the pad for several hours.

This means that the unpleasant odor that many women have experienced when using disposable pads is not from their bodily fluids. It's from the mixture of their bodily fluids with the chemicals in the disposable pads.

Pain-Free Periods: Yes, It Is Possible!

I'm still kind of in shock about this whole thing. Think about it. If you cut your finger, does the blood from your finger smell badly? No. Is it gross? No.

Ladies, we are not gross, and neither is anything that our bodies were created to do. Although the devil would love for us to hate the process that enables us to reproduce, he is simply jealous because we can do something that he can't.

I began realizing how much we as women have rejected, hated, and loathed our periods. The products we have been using have contributed to this. I believe that many women are using products during their periods that their bodies want to reject and are rejecting.

I also believe from my own experience that these products were enabling and increasing the pain that I was experiencing.

The disposable products that I had used for years had helped me reject and stay disconnected from what my body was trying to naturally do. Wow. It always amazes me what else God changes my mind about. I never would have guessed that there was anything negative connected to the products that I had been using for so long.

Getting Pain-Free

Men, I hope that you will share this information with the women in your lives.

As I type this, I'm loving my body more. I'm so much freer today than I was yesterday.

There are some new things involved with cloth pads, but it's more than worth any adjustments that I've made. The ones that I bought have cloth wings that wrap around the undergarment and snap together to stay in place. They are machine washable, machine dryable, and reusable.

After using the cloth pad, I simply fold it in half with the clean side on the outside and the used side on the inside and then put it in a plastic zippered bag in my purse.

I put my used cloth pads in a gallon-sized plastic bag at home until the end of my period. Then, I wash all of them in a separate load in the washing machine. After drying them in the dryer, I put them in a new, gallon-sized plastic bag and store them for the next month. This has only been a small adjustment.

The pads are supposed to last for years. This makes sense because you only use them approximately 12 times per year.

I've found that using cloth pads is actually more discreet than using disposable products. I don't have to go down that aisle in the store anymore or feel strange at the checkout counter. There are also no noisy wrappers to deal with or any used products to throw away in public or home bathrooms.

I also don't use as many pads now that I use cloth pads and am more in tune with my body. I no longer fight what my body was made to do. When I go to the restroom, I take an extra minute or two and leave my body "open" and stay in a posture of urinating even once I am done urinating.

I give my body some time to release what is there. During the time that my body releases the most during my period, I tend to go to the restroom probably every 1-2 hours to give my body a chance to release what it needs to in the toilet. I really don't have much that is released into the cloth pad unless I am unable to get to a restroom for a long period of time. It's interesting that I never even thought to do this for more than 20 years until I switched to cloth pads.

I am able to use just one thick, cloth pad overnight with no problem and with no restroom breaks. So, you will have no problem with cloth pads if you are in a situation where you are unable to have frequent restroom breaks.

Getting Pain-Free

I can't imagine ever going back to disposable products after using all-natural, cloth pads. I actually appreciate and love my body more now since I changed the products that I was using.

My joy, confidence, and understanding of my identity have been positively affected through this change. I'm no longer in a mode of self-rejection, shame, or misery for one week every month.

I can't contain my excitement about this revelation. I'm already thinking of a friend that I know who has had such horrible pain during her cycle that she has often had to stay home from work. Anyone been there? I have, but thank God, no more!

Say out loud, "No more period pain!"

What is sad about this is that I suffered needlessly for over two decades. I won't anymore though, and you don't have to either.

It has now been more than three years since I switched to cloth pads. I haven't once taken any pain medication during my period for over three years! Some months, I forget how bad the pain used to be. Other months, the pain has attempted to come back.

When the pain tried to come back, I

Pain-Free Periods: Yes, It Is Possible!

simply repeated the steps that I mentioned before. I don't accept the pain. I also do not come into agreement with it. I do not allow it to come back. I resist it; I stand up to it, and it leaves.

I've also learned that our bodies react to what we put on them and in them. The foods that we eat are important. Junk foods, processed foods, and sugar that isn't naturally in foods are not good things to eat or drink especially when a woman has her period. Overeating can also contribute to pain. It's also good to drink a lot of water. This helps flush things out of your system. These are some of the lessons that I've learned. Treat your body well. Put good things in it and on it.

What are you putting in your body?

We have authority and power over pain. We must actually use the authority though in order for it to benefit us.

What do you need to use your authority over?

What change are you going to make today?

What do you need to stop claiming that you have?

How is God leading you after reading this? What is your next step?

Getting Pain-Free

What truth have you learned? How are you going to use what you've learned?

Who will you share this with today?

Living pain-free: it is possible! What are you waiting for?

Helpful Scripture References:

1. "For God so loved the world that He gave His only begotten Son, that whoever believes in Him should not perish but have everlasting life. For God did not send His Son into the world to condemn the world, but that the world through Him might be saved" (John 3:16-17, NKJV).
2. "And do not be conformed to this world, but be transformed by the renewing of your mind, that you may prove what is that good and acceptable and perfect will of God" (Romans 12:2, NKJV).
3. "And you He made alive, who were dead in trespasses and sins, in which you once walked according to the course of this world, according to the prince of the power of the air, the spirit who now works in the sons of disobedience" (Ephesians 2:1-2, NKJV).
4. "For you were bought at a price; therefore glorify God in your body and in your spirit, which are God's" (I Corinthians 6:20, NKJV).

Other titles by this author:

I Found God Outside of Church

Stolen Identity